The Battle for Sanity

Want to know what a battle for sanity is....
Imagine a battlefield, with your obviously different sides. Both fighting for what they think is "peace. "
Imagine the chaos, the turmoil, the pain. Now imagine all of this is going on inside of your head where there is no escape. You can't hide in a ditch till the fighting is over. All you can do is plow through the very middle hoping to stop it before it reaches pure destruction. Just hoping for one second the battle would stop and you could rest.

Hello there, my name is Tiffany and I suffer from mental illness. Everyday of my life is a constant battle inside my head. Every day there is a new battle between sane and insane. Every single day a struggle between staying alive and ending my life. Mental illness is not talked about in these times. No one takes it seriously. But for those of us who go through that constant battle we know how real it is.

In this book I hope to show you how to survive, how to keep going even when you feel like giving up. How to not only manage this, but to survive it.

In doing so I hope to let others know that they are not alone. That there are people like them. And we get it. We understand. And we are here for you.

This book is a collection of poems I've written beginning when I was twelve. Some of them are dark. Some of them are cute and funny. But all of them stem from a personal experience I've gone through.

So my content warning is this. There will be things that might trigger you, upset you, make you cry. Just know it is not my intent to offend anyone. And I hope after reading this you feel a sense of belonging.

You are loved,
You are wanted,
You are needed in this life,
You are strong
And you can survive this.

Your beautiful disaster
Tiffany.

Let's start with what I call the 5 steps to survival. These are steps I've learned to help get through anything that life throws at you.

Step one: Trauma
You must go through some type of trauma. Doesn't matter how big or small. If it affects your moods then it is enough to be considered trauma. You must be broken before you can heal.

Step two: Anger
Get angry. Get mad. But get angry in a healthy way. Don't self destruct. Go buy a set of cheap plates and smash them, go to a batting cage and swing away. Get angry.

Step three: Sadness
Now it's time to be sad. Release all that anger, the hurt, everything step one made you feel, let it out. Bottling up emotions can seriously damage your mental health. Cry it out. Let those emotions flow.

Step four: Acceptance
Accept what happened. Learn from it. Just remember the lessons learned from step one. And never repeat it again.

Step five: Recovery
Reflect on the previous steps, what you learned, how you felt, what you went through, and move on. Holding on to hate and anger will only hurt you in the end. Move on and find your happiness. I promise you it's out there.

There's no time limit on how long these steps take. Take every single second you need, and never let someone make you feel bad for how you deal with your trauma.

Chapter one: The early years.

Ah, the early years...

These are different for some. I'd say my early years started around the age of 12. That's when I wrote my first poem. When I figured out I could actually create something.

I was an awkward child, didn't really fit in. Wasn't girly, but wasn't a tomboy either. I spent a lot of time alone.

So I started writing. I wrote everything down in journals.

At 13 I experienced my first trauma.

I was raped...

I know some of you know that trauma, and I'm so sorry you do.
I also know some of you don't know that trauma, and I'm so thankful you don't.

I was broken. I didn't understand. I didn't tell anyone, not even my mom. I was ashamed and scared. I wasn't supposed to be where I was. My mother had warned me not to go there. But I didn't listen. And I was afraid of getting in trouble.

Later that year I was diagnosed with Bi-Polar type 1.... I didn't know anything about it. At that time there wasn't the Internet with endless articles about it. No one talked about it. Until I was diagnosed I didn't even know there was such a thing as mental illness.

My mother was in disbelief. She didn't believe the doctors. But then again she still didn't know what had happened to me. So she just blamed it on hormones. Because of my silence I went untreated.
In this chapter you'll be able to see the downfall of my sanity. As I was trying to cope and understand what was going on inside my head.. Why I couldn't control my moods and what led to my first cutting experience.

This is a group of poems from my early years...

I hope you enjoy them.

Your beautiful disaster
Tiffany

The Beginning

For you to heal
You must first break

So break,
Shatter,
Implode

Then put yourself together
The way you want to be

Pick yourself up
Pull if you have to

Move forward
Then be free

RAPE ME

Whip me now
Lick me up and down
Till I lose every frown
Slice my fragile skin
Till we engage unseen sin
Pull my hair while we both are bare
Tie my arms to separated desires
Shackle my ankles
Take my movement powers
Shred my attire
Let it drop to the floor
Choking grip at my throat
Lights off shut the door
Leather straps across my back
Make me weak
"RAPE ME"

News

The news of your passing
Tightens in my chest
My heart feels empty and lost

You were not deserving
Of such fate
Though it was sealed at birth

Fly free
I'll see you in the next life.

Death of the fae

The world is watching
as my wings unfurl
The world is watching
the death of a girl
The world is watching
as I begin to cry
The world is watching
as I slowly die

If I would have known

My heart feels like a black hole tonight
This is something I can't bare
The only thing that runs through my mind
Is the time we would share
We used to be everything
Just like the perfect dream
But someone didn't want us together
So it would seem
I even changed everything
Just so you could be mine
Maybe I should have realized this
And done it at a better time
Maybe it was the stars, the time, or the weather
But something didn't want me happy
No one wanted us to be together
Our last night together
Man what a time
Sometimes I wish I could stop and rewind
If I had known it was our last walk down the street
I would have looked into your eyes
And not at my feet.
I would have taken in every moment with you
Because this pain I feel is so untrue

If I would have known it would be our last kiss
I wish I would have known
Because it's something I miss
If I had known it would be our last hug
Believe me babe I wouldn't have let go
And my feelings for you I would have let show
And if I had known you were going to die
I would have told you then and I wouldn't have to cry
And if your looking down
Watching me write this
Know that when I was with you
I was in perpetual bliss
Each day I must face this is true
To this day I still love you.

Chapter 2

The trauma years

These were probably the worst years of my life.
So much happened in such a short amount of time. My traumatic years lasted 12 years. That goes to show you there's no time limit for these. It has to play out and has to happen on its own time.

I lost a love,
I lost many friends,
I lost my uncle,
I lost my aunt,
I lost my daughter,
I lost my mother,
And I lost myself.

But in all this loss I found my true friends, I found my strength, and I began to find myself.

You must go through trauma(no matter how big or small) to be able to heal from what broke you.

But the beauty in breaking is you can put your pieces back together the way you want. You get to decide how you heal.

The Loss

The pain is unbearable
The tears sting as they flow
A once closed wound
Now opened once more
I thought that I was done
That I had healed
But the pain has returned
Much stronger than before
This isn't fair!
This is not how it was supposed to be
A loving heart stopped beating
A warm touch forever gone
A soft voice no longer heard
A caring mother taken to soon
A family left in pieces
Not knowing what to do
A shattered life of broken trust
Never to be made whole

A wound that is open
Never to gully close
Years of pain
Is now at peace
Rest easy momma
Love follows in your place.

Statistic

Death is easy
Its life that's hard

Bruised and broken
I'm standing on the edge
I'm ashamed to look at
myself in the mirror
Your loving touch
Turned to the violent hands
That left me this way
There is nothing left of me
An empty shell that once
Housed a strong spirit
A hallow memory of the woman
I once was
Looking down from my
Unsteady perch

Wondering...
Will it hurt?
Of course it will
The pain from falling
Will end quickly
The shattering of a
Once vibrant soul
Will be felt by everyone
I ever knew
One little step
Is all its going to take
Why do I hesitate?
Why do I think someone
Will try and save me?
I've waited long enough
Time to go
A blackened heart
A broken soul
All at once
Will be no more
Eyes closed
Tears flowing
Heart racing
Blood rushing
For the very last time
To bad
Its just another suicide...

Burdened

Buried under the crushing weight of my decisions.
Your constant glare forever burned into the rough skin on my neck

Being one step ahead of your lies seems impossible
Why must you do this?
Why must you be so afraid to love me?
Your touch
cared of what we are
You're scared to come home
Our souls dance when our eyes meet
We tremble as we touch
Your water calms the ever burning fire inside of me
My black broken heart still longs for your embrace
As a stream of tears flow
I ask myself why
As I sit at my window
Forever waiting for your return
Waiting for you to walk through the door
Waiting for you to take me in your arms
My lips crashing into yours
The weight of your body is the only comfort that calms me
But it's your choices that have put me here
Your constant neglect that has driven the love from my heart
Your lack of care that has opened my eyes to your true self
I will force myself to forgive you
I end this battle bruised and broken
My eyes opened to your fake smile
Your lying words
Your empty touch
Never again will you use me
Never again will you fool me
Never again will your tears move me to action
The bridge is burnt
The pain no longer there
You have lost your control of me
I love you
But now I let you go.

Empty

8th grade
What a year
Lots of drugs
Lots of beer

Late night
Skating rink
Now I don't
Want to think

There you were
Standing there
Here I was
Chewing on my hair

Coming over
To say please
Stay with me all night
Never leave hold tight

Walking home
All alone
Falling rain
So cold

16 golden age
Car coming
Drunken rage

At school
Empty hall
At home
Phone call

There you were
Now your dead
Here I am
Eyes burning red

Now tell me
How I'm supposed
To make it through
This useless life
Without you.

What have I done...

What have I done to myself again
I've let myself get my hopes up
And in return
Receive nothing
A few words
Nothing for the days that follow

He tells me he loves me
But if he did
Could he go so long
Without a word

My heart bleeds
At the thought
Of not having him
My body aches
At the thought
Of his soft touch

The roughness
Of his scars
Make me want to
Hold on tighter

Am I ready for this again?
My heart can't take anymore...

Reckless

Time and time again
I run towards the danger
Knowing the outcome
I still follow the same path
Forever sealing the darkness
That calls toy soul
Time after time
I'm reckless

Whole

As I sit in the dark abyss
You put me in
Crying
Wondering why I wasn't

Good enough
Why was it so easy
For you to discard me
Like I didn't matter
Replaying every single
Memory of us
Wishing I knew
What I did wrong
Will I ever feel whole?

Raindrop

The rain falls
Mimicking the tears
The pain flows
As swiftly as a river
Through a shattered barrier
For that's what I've become,
Shattered
Never to drift ashore
Set in motion by
The power of the memories
Drowning in the water
Never to rise above
Forever adrift in purgatory

Deadly

Just like the poison apple
He knew she was dangerous
But he couldn't deny her beauty
And taste
He knew she would kill him..

Plague

I should have known this
Happiness wouldn't last
The darkness is creeping
In again
How can I fight this plague
Why can't I end this battle
I wish the happiness would stay

Lies

Lies upon lies
You try to destroy me
Try to take away how far I've come
Lies upon lies
You try and break me
But I'm not her anymore
And I'll win in the end
Hope you like the bed
You must now lie in

Release

After all this time it's still you...

You've come back again, not in person.
No you wouldn't do that...
My memory is all I have.
But you won't leave...
You crawl around like an insect.
Leaving behind the what ifs...
The thoughts that plague me,
Have the power to cripple my body...
My chest tightens.
My heart bleeds...
And slowly my light dims.
This is the end of this...
I release the damn memories.
       I release you....

Smother me

Your love is smothering me
I can't breathe
My chest has tightened
As my soul begins to leave
The air has left my lungs
Soon my body will follow

Chaotic Mind

A chaotic mind that won't stay calm
Why can't I silence the thoughts plaguing
My every waking moment?
Just dont think about it they say....
Yeah, if it were only that easy
I tried to subdue the manic thoughts
But just like an insect they creep
Back in
Leaving behind thoughts of self destruction
Be happy they say,
How can I?
I'm left remembering how dark and
Hopeless this world can be
Just relax they tell me
But how can I relax when

My chest feels as if it will implode
In on itself
I wish they could understand
I'm glad they don't live with
This constant struggle
I wish they knew how envious of
Them I am
A chaotic mind forever racing
A tired body just wanting to rest
The two together
I am a beautiful mess.

Once again you have come back
Saying things that I want to hear

Am I stupid for still wanting you?
Am I crazy for still missing you?
I do this to myself
Over and over
Expecting a different outcome
Each time
You're late
I promised myself I wouldn't
Watch for you this time
Yet, here I am
Looking out my door
Waiting for you to come
Letting my heart get my
Hopes up once again
The fire is burning out of control
I fear it may consume me
But why should I have to hide my
Passion for you
Why am I not good enough for you?
You say give you time..
But what if today is all we have?
What do I need to do to make you see?
That no matter how many times you
Lie to me
Disappoint me
And no matter how many people
Try and poison me against you
That my love for you will never leave
My want of you will never fade
My picture of happiness will haunt
The walls of my mind until
I fade from this earth
It's you
It will always be you

I can't wait forever
But I will never love as I love you
I will wait...
Just hope you aren't too late.

Chapter 3. The Recovery Years

Finally we have reached the recovery years. It took along
time for me to get here and that's ok.
You may reach yours before I did
and if you do, that's awesome and I'm proud of you.

These years are not all joy filled either,
but in this chapter I hope you see my rise to regain
sanity, regain my self, and most importantly
my survival…

For you

A soul awakening
From a decade long rest
Do I trust this feeling?
Last time I did
It ended badly
I was ripped apart
But you have me feeling
Whole again
I'm scared
And like a child
I wish to hide
But I'll push through
This fear
And face
The unknown
    For you I will
           Teenage love

Romantic eyes

Toned hips
Top it off
With perfect lips
I want a guy
With a heart of gold
Who will be with me
Till we grow old
I want a guy
Who will help me clean
And won't run away
When I am mean
I want a guy
Who will laugh when I fall
And treat me like a princess
At my very own ball
He'll bring me flowers
He'll bring me candy
He'll say strange things
And take me to beaches that are sandy
He'll write poems
And sing me to sleep
And when I've had a bad day
He'll rub my feet
He'll always know
The right words to say
And never touch me
In a violent way
He'll treat me right
And never wrong
And when I ask
He'll buy me a new bong
He'll massage my back
And rub my head
And won't pressure me to do

Anything but sleep in a bed
Now I know this is a lot to ask
And it's a very big task
But I want a guy who will
Do all of the above
Then I will have found my love

New beginning

Cold winter nights
Warm summer air
Nature in raw form
We both are bare

Late nights
Music so loud
Two of us together
Feeling proud

Early mornings
Chaos everywhere
Only two people
Stop and stare

Loving hearts
Thriving souls
Two simple people
Now are one

Burning

Like the lamb to the lion
I'm drawn to the danger
The ever burning fire
Ignites at every turn
A ball of warmth to hot
To ignore
To ignore it would be as if
I was denying who I was
Deep inside
Why must I burn?
Why can't it be calmed?
Can I never be anything
But destruction…

Mistakes

The mistakes I've made have lead
Me to where I am today

The choices forever on my soul
My skin bares the marks of my life
Blaming everyone
But myself

My mistakes
My choices
My life
My disaster

You

A question that's always asked
"Who is this you"
Let me tell you about this "you"

He is the man that makes me feel whole
He is the man that can calm me
With just his touch
He is the man that makes me
A priority
He is the man that cares for me,
Looks after me,
Protects me,
Believes in me,
And can make me smile with
Just a simple smirk
The one who loves me with
Everything he has
And the one I never
Want to let go

So if you're still wondering
"Who this you is"
Take a glance in the mirror
For you are him.

Paper heart

I love you

Three little words
That holds more
Meaning than you
Could ever know
Please don't stop
My paper heart might bleed

Butterflies

The butterflies have awakened
Inside of me again
Little flutters of hope
Tiny wings making me feel
Alive again
Small little movements that
Make my heart beat faster
With every touch
Growing anticipation for
What's to come
I hope these butterflies
Are real this time
That I'm not getting
My hopes up
Just to be let down
Please….
Let these butterflies grow
            Am I?

Is this happiness

Or is it a façade
I hide behind?

Am I truly becoming who
I was meant to be,
Or am I just making
Myself into what others
Want me to be?

Have I arrived to
The "adult"
Destination required
Of someone

Is it time to accept my
Place in this world?

Am I ready for that?

Misleading

I need to tell you something
And this I can not bare
It has to do with you pulling
On my long beautiful hair
Now when you get it wet
From the scalp down
To the tip,
I swear sometimes
I can feel it rip
As you lather me up
From my head down
To my toes
I think from here you
Know where this goes
From the scratches
And the cries
You wipe my teary eyes
And as you grab a towel
So you can dry me off
If you touch me
I promise
I'm very soft
Now all of this happened
While we were in the tub
And as I calm down
My tummy is what you'll rub
Now let me give you this
Crazy little fact
Doesn't it sound sexy,
When you give your cat a bath

I hoped you liked it and I hope beyond all reason that it has brought you some sort of comfort.
If you laughed, cried, thought of something that had happened, or just tore through it, I'm glad

You took the time to read it.

And if you read it because you needed it, I really hope it helped you.

Remember loves

You are wanted
You matter
You are needed in this life
And you have survived every bad day in your life.
I'm so very proud of you all.
You are true warriors.

As always

Your beautiful disaster
Tiffany

www.ingramcontent.com/pod-product-compliance
Lightning Source LLC
Chambersburg PA
CBHW071200220526
45468CB00003B/1089